Dementia:
My
Journey as a
Caregiver

Dementia:
My
Journey as a
Caregiver

SUMMER

Rev. date: 03/24/2023

To order additional copies of this book, contact:
Xlibris
844-714-8691
www.Xlibris.com
Orders@Xlibris.com
781428

ACKNOWLEDGEMENTS

I want to give thanks to my family, especially to my Aunti, and her eldest daughter as well as to my friends. You all have help mom and me in more ways than I can express. Thank You for loving my mom and being so selfless!

Introduction

Dementia is a general term for loss of memory and other mental abilities severe enough to interfere with daily life. It is caused by physical changes in the brain.

Dementia, in my opinion is a new term for memory loss, or "that stuff" as my auntie always says. It means that a person has been given a terminal diagnosis. It is progressive and sometimes causes problems with their thinking, behavior, and eventually their ability to function normally on their own. It is a terminal disease. According to Ford-Martin, dementia in itself is not a disease but a syndrome; its symptoms are common to several brain diseases. (P. Ford-Martin 2020)- reviewed medically by Jennifer Casarella, MD 2020

I am writing this book as my way of doing self - therapy. I am constantly reminded of just how much a part of my life including spending time with my mom. As I look back over the years we spent together, fishing, picking peas and veggies, going to church functions, and laughing at many things that had happened, to name a few things. We really enjoyed ourselves together. I truly miss her.

Mom's Diagnosis

My mom was diagnosed with Dementia in 2015, three years prior to this she had called me while I was living in Georgia, asking me to come home to California because she really needed me to help take care of her. I laughingly said, "Mom, you are good, you can take care of yourself". I didn't know that she REALLY DID NEED ME, and it was just a matter of time before it would be revealed, just how much.

When she was tested, she had failed the horribly put together testing mechanism that the administrator gave to her. One test consisted of drawing a clock and putting in the numbers correctly around it; another test: she was told five things that she was asked to remember in the order that it was given to her approximately five minutes prior; lastly, she was given a diagram and told to draw it. What I found disturbing, was that some of those things would be difficult for anyone to do. I looked at her struggling and told her not to worry too much about it because I couldn't do some of it either. That was to make her feel better, although, I was being truthful.

My mom, nor I weren't given anything to encourage or inspire her to strengthen her brain. She felt bad and started to cry, I started to cry, and my younger brother just sat there. She wasn't given any literature to prepare for anything. No puzzles, no exercises that may encourage her to think. Even her neurologist didn't offer anything but medications, that of course had its side affects. Obviously, I would have preferred that the doctors had given my mom options for increasing her brain activity. When the different therapists finally started coming to see her, there wasn't much brain therapy going on at all. A guy came out to do walking therapy, another lady therapist came to work on her strengthening her arms. She actually enjoyed the male therapist visits, especially when he brought her fruit from his trees in his backyard.

I used to tell different people that my mom was walking like a "Negro slave." Instead of picking up her feet, she would shuffle her feet. When she visited her family on the East Coast, they finally understood what I was saying. One of my aunts asked me, "What is wrong with your mother?"

I really didn't know all the questions to ask and felt like I was and still am learning things by trial and error. It appeared to me that as soon as mom was given the diagnosis, she began to say what she couldn't do any more. She couldn't open her bag/purse to put things in it, she couldn't write very well (this she had already noticed beforehand), she would tell others as well as myself, "You know I have Dementia". I would laugh sometimes and tell her that she should still do whatever the Lord has blessed her with to be able to do for herself, while she was still able to do so. I would only do things for her that I knew she wasn't able to do. This wasn't exactly what she wanted to hear, but I was actually following the instructions of the social worker coupled with my own common sense.

She was later told that she shouldn't cook anymore, although for a while she still was able to do so. One thing that I really am on the fence about is that, it seems to me that maybe the doctors should talk to the caregiver, family members, etc., about the diagnosis before telling the patient, because in her case, she seemed to decline more after hearing what was wrong with her. I felt like she had just succumbed to the knowledge that she was losing her mind. This thought was making me feel angry. I wanted her to fight for her own self- preservation. Just because the "doctor" tells you something, in my opinion, it doesn't make it so. There are so many other things that can be done to prevent or at least slow down the process- without taking the prescription pills! Which are truly killing you anyway!

One day, I decided to reach out to two of my siblings. These were on two separate calls, first to my sister and then to my youngest brother, asking for them to come over and do something – anything with mom at least once a week. They both replied, "Once a week!" One would have thought it was rehearsed since it was stated exactly that same way and with the same tone. I was too tired to do or feel anything but disgust. I have never asked them that question again. I was being pulled emotionally, mentally, and then physically in so many directions.

At this time, as an Early Childhood Substitute Teacher. I was on call and I had to stop accepting assignments so I could take my mom to her appointments. I was living off my savings for the first year and a half, until I was able with the help my friend Lucy, to get her the "overrated Share of Cost" down to zero, and only then, was I able to get paid to take care of mom through the state ran In Home Supportive Services, better known as IHSS. Once that was revealed, my siblings really felt that I was "supposed to do everything", their verbal thoughts: "because you are being paid for that – Whatever "THAT" was supposed to be". I really knew then, that I was alone in this journey. They didn't care that it was their mom also and no matter what, one person would never be able to give the proper care to anyone 24/7, that is just impossible. The funny thing is that I wasn't being paid 24/7, as they seemed to believe, to take care of all her needs. When you receive funds from the In-Home Supportive Services Department, they send out a social worker to access the needs of the person needing the services. This can go from washing them up in the morning through the total needs of the day, ending in putting them to bed. Each thing that is done is accrued in minutes. She would always ask me, "how long does it take to do this?" It was very frustrating because, I had to start thinking in terms of minutes, while I'm trying to take care of my mom. The worker would tell me, that she can only figure out the pay, based on how long it took for each need to be taken care of. The pay has a cap on it, so everything you may do, isn't going to be paid for. So, my point here is that no matter what I was getting paid, it wasn't for the 24-hour period of her care – and that's point the agency expressed to me.

I know in my heart of hearts that I did what I could, the best way I could for mom and I find extreme comfort with that. It would have been so much easier and nicer for my mom, if the whole family had pitched in with loving, helpful hands. I have spoken to many people during this journey, and they all said the same thing – Gurl, it's always just one or two that will come and take care of their loved one, even if it's a large family. I was kind of shocked to hear this. You know, it's ALWAYS someone out there that has had, or is dealing with the same thing you are, which is why it's important to share your stories.

I thank God for my Aunti, who was very instrumental in assisting me whenever she could. Understand me, this woman is three years older than my mom, but because of her love for her sister from another mother, who couldn't be closer if they had been raised in the same household. I've known this woman for sixty-one of my almost 66 years on this earth. I love her dearly. I was taught creative things to do with my hands, from her that I still use today.

When she was available, Aunti would accommodate my mom and me whenever there was a need for mom to go to an appointment, if I wasn't able to do it. When you join the "senior club" and find yourself with less and less friends still living, or friends that are no longer able to get around, life can be very lonely. I tried to keep my mom interested in doing things to keep her spirits up, such as joining one of the Oakland Senior Centers where she was able to exercise to music and meet other interesting seniors. This is something that she really enjoyed.

Sometimes, we went to a neighboring Catholic Church for a fun filled outing that included food and music, and mom truly enjoyed this because eating, dancing and listening to some good o' music was something mom has always enjoyed.

One day, I drove down to Porterville, CA, which is approximately 4 hours away, with mom and Aunti in tow. This was so mom could spend some quality time with her older brother and wife. She stayed there for one week. It seemed like that week just flew by, before I realized it, my uncle was calling me to let me know what time he would be bringing her back home. If I'm to be honest, I wasn't ready to receive her back so soon, but it was my responsibility, so I rushed to meet them at my Aunti's place, after my day at work.

This visit was an eye opener for her brother and his wife, who had now gotten a bird's eye view of what I was dealing with. This is why I wanted her to visit other family members and friends, because until she does, no one really understands what I'm speaking about, or going through.

As time went by, mom seemed content in watching her TV programs such as: The Wendy Williams Show, The Real, Harry, Ellen, the Lifetime channel as well as LMN, Dancing with the Stars, and LOVED watching "her baby" Curry with the Golden State Warriors! I would have loved for her to have been able to meet him in person. She would walk daily to visit her neighbors in the building that she lived in to have breakfast, coffee, or just to vent. I became concerned that she began to spend more and more of her day watching TV, versus trying to exercise her legs and arms. I found that if I didn't do these things with her, she wasn't interested. When I questioned her, she would say, "You ain't always here, you don't know what I do!" When her therapist came over, she would lie and tell them that she was exercising every day.

The eldest of my two brothers was home with mom on this particular day. This brother wasn't around much, and I told him previously that the woman you last saw, will not be the same woman, when you see her again. As I had predicted, he was devastated when he walked in and saw her. I later found him in tears, because he couldn't believe that his mom was not able to do the things he had been used to seeing her do. One day I came home to a funny situation, he was in the kitchen, cracking up laughing, stating that mom was in the living room with the physical therapist telling lies about how she has been exercising every day! I immediately went in the room and told the therapist that she was not telling the truth and we all, including mom, began laughing so hard, tears were coming. That was one of our lighter moments.

There were times when she would get angry and ball her fists up at me! She was spoiled and when I didn't do everything she wanted me to do, this would be one of things she would do, then I would tell her, she better not do that. She would then look at me, and then walk back into her living room area to sit down. This happened rarely though. Other times, I would hear her crying and it was very hard for me to listen to this. I would try to discern if she was trying to get attention, if she was hurting, or feeling upset or angry about her situation. This would bring out all types of emotions. During the meetings I would attend to help me understand the journey, I would hear that these things are to be expected. It reminded me of when I worked with the special need's population, because I would feel these same kind of feelings – sometimes I would be crying right with them and now it's happening with mom.

When mom would act out, yelling, or complaining, I felt the need to remind her that I am only one person, and that she actually has four children, and maybe she should call one of them to help out. She would always reply, **"They aren't going to come."** Unfortunately, she was mostly right about that, which is why I stated that I'm in this journey all alone. That's a horrible feeling to have, because caregiving is a 24-hour job that I didn't apply for. I truly felt trapped, unloved, uncared for by my own family, who I have helped whenever they needed me, especially the youngest two siblings.

Now, what I have noticed is that even when people see her and spend time with her, they are in denial of what is really going on. Different ones would think that she could do things that she really couldn't do. When you're not around a person with Dementia a lot, or don't have any experience with someone with the disease, it can be difficult to come to grips with the fact that this person that you once knew, is no longer that same person anymore. Things that you were accustomed to seeing them do, they can't do anymore and sometimes you may believe that the person with Dementia is faking the funk. In other words, they are playing you. Now, there have been times that I was feeling that way, and I was there every day caring for her. In my opinion, she would do things when others came around that she stated she couldn't or didn't want to do when it was just her and myself. I felt she would be showing off for her audience.

As time went on, it was obvious to me and others that she wasn't able to do simple things, such as, eat her food without dropping or spilling it. When I look back in time, I remembered seeing some indicators when we would go out to eat, she would always complain about getting food on her clothes. I really didn't think much of it at the time though. She would also leave her purse or cell phone on the bus, but was truly blessed, because she would get a call from the bus driver or agent, stating that they found the lost item(s), but now I know these things were some early signs of her dementia.

According to the doctors that I have spoken to, Alzheimer's patients will also become bedridden towards the end, which can increase their risk of having fatal blood clots, The doctors that I have spoken to, including the neurologist mentioned that Alzheimer's disease is the sixth-leading cause of death in the United States.

Myth: **Alzheimer's** disease is not **fatal**. Reality: **Alzheimer's** disease has no survivors. It destroys brain cells and causes memory changes, erratic behaviors and loss of body functions.

Some examples: My mom, lost the ability to hold her own utensils correctly, couldn't make it to the toilet in time, couldn't wash herself up, brush her teeth correctly, and her gait was affected. The latter was something I was troubled with and one of the reasons I made a doctor's appointment for her to be seen and tested.

I wanted to share this information because it would be beneficial for those of us who are, has or will be a caregiver of a loved one and also feel victimized by the overwhelming circumstances one finds themselves in, and feeling like there's no favorable way out. Below are some things that may help you prepare if you will "for the process." These are the stages of loss that I witnessed with my mom.

Stage 1: No Impairment – Normal Outward Behavior

During this stage, Alzheimer's disease is not detectable, and no memory problems or other symptoms of dementia are evident. *There are symptoms, but because we, laypersons are unaware of what to look for, we really don't know it's there. It could be a few years before you will see anything of significance.*

Stage 2: Lightly Declining

The senior may notice minor memory problems or lose things around the house, although not to the point where the memory loss can easily be distinguished from normal age-related memory loss. The person will still do well on memory tests and the disease is unlikely to be detected by physicians or loved ones.

I could surmise that my mom knew something was amiss based on a conversation I had with her approximately 4-5 years before her diagnosis. She called me when I lived in Georgia in 2011, stating that she needed me to come back to California and help her. I told her that she didn't really need me, and she would be alright without me. I just thought that this was another way for her to get me back to California, to be with her; but she knew something wasn't right within herself.

Stage 3: Mild Declining

At this stage, the friends and family members of the senior may begin to notice memory and cognitive problems. Performance on memory and cognitive tests are affected and physicians will be able to detect impaired cognitive function.

Patients in stage 3 will have difficulty in many areas including:

- finding the right word during conversations
- remembering names of new acquaintances
- planning and organizing
- forgetting something they've just read

People with stage three Alzheimer's may also frequently lose personal possessions, including valuables.

I can't truly determine if it was due to simple forgetfulness, or the beginning stages of dementia. This disease is not really textbook, because doctors are still doing research, and I have found that they, the doctors are still experimenting on their patients. This is where I believe the term, "Practicing Physicians originally came from, because the doctors are practicing on us, the patients. Every person doesn't experience this horrible disease the same way. Yes, there are some similarities, but definitely not exact.

Stage 4: Moderately Declining

In stage four of Alzheimer's disease clear cut symptoms of Alzheimer's disease are apparent. Patients with stage four Alzheimer's disease:

- Have difficulty with simple arithmetic
- May forget details about their life histories
- Have poor short term memory (may not recall what they ate for breakfast, for example)
- Inability to manage finance and pay bills

My mom never like to do things such as, manage her checking account, so it is hard for me to decipher if and when this stage applies to her. These examples didn't apply until now in 2017.

Stage 5: Moderately Severe Declining

During the fifth stage of Alzheimer's, patients begin to need help with many day-to-day activities. People in stage five of the disease may experience:

- Significant confusion
- Inability to recall simple details about themselves such as their own phone number
- Difficulty dressing appropriately

Note: The above is true for my mom. I started noticing her inability to bathe herself correctly in 2016. She was still able to toilet independently, but always complained of vaginal dryness, which the doctors stated came with getting older. There were many times she complained of being constipated. I tried to encourage her to drink more water, purchase stool softeners, and prune juice. Although, this was another thing that came back to bite me, because, once these things started working, then she would accuse me of giving her that stuff that made her bowels loose. I just couldn't win!

On the other hand, patients in stage five maintain a modicum of functionality. They typically can still bathe and toilet independently. They're able to still be able recognize their family members and some details about their personal histories, especially their childhood and youth.

Stage 6: Severe Declining

Patients with the sixth stage of Alzheimer's disease need constant supervision and frequently require professional care. Symptoms can include:

- Confusion or unawareness of environment and surroundings
- Major personality changes and potential behavior problems
- The need for assistance with activities of daily living such as toileting and bathing
- Inability to recognize faces except closest friends and relatives
- Inability to remember most details of personal history
- Loss of bowel and bladder control
- Wandering

Again, this stage isn't an exact science for my mom. A lot of these stages aren't always typical. This was evident with mom in early 2017. One thing is though, she never wandered anywhere, and she definitely still recognized her children, grands and great grands, including Punchy, the great grand dog. She loves singing with me when I came over to polish her nails during our frequent visits at her nursing home. I would bring my Bluetooth speaker and play Motown sounds, or gospel music. She would be soooo happy, talking crap in between, remembering things or people as we all do when we hear a certain song.

Stages 7: Very Severe Decline

Stage seven is the final stage of Alzheimer's disease. Because Alzheimer's disease is a *terminal illness*. Patients in stage seven are nearing death. In stage seven of the disease, patients lose ability to respond to their environment or communicate. While they may still be able to utter words and phrases, they have no insight into their condition and need assistance with all activities of daily living. In the final stages of the illness, patients may lose their ability to swallow.

Note: Please know that once my mom was diagnosed with this disease, she began a steady decline. Some things that she would do before, she immediately stated that she could no longer do them anymore. An example of this is, I would say to her, "mom what happened, why can't you put this into your purse?" She would answer, "You know I have dementia." I felt like she started using her diagnosis as a way to get me and others to do things that she really didn't want to deal with. I hate this disease so much, for so many reasons. It takes a person dignity, it destroys relationships, it attacks the care person's judgment; meaning the care person finds themselves in a place of aloneness, feelings of abandonment, not knowing if they are doing the right things for their loved one(s), its just not a good place to be. It can actually be paralleled with the "Devil", whose God-given job is to "Kill, Steal, and Destroy!", and that's what this horrible disease has done for my mom and me. It has destroyed my joy of seeing my mom dance, cook, eat her favorite foods, to do simple things like hold her great grands, have simple conversations, come to my classroom and read books to my students, etc... I know people grow old and start losing their abilities to do certain things, but I believe that she is too young to have to endure this "Thing" that has change our lives forever.

On my to work this day, I noticed that my mom's big toe was looking swollen and dark. I immediately became concerned, especially since she was diabetic. The first thing that came across my mind was ***"amputation."*** I remember crying all the way to work, not knowing how to handle this new situation. I couldn't just call in at the last minute, so I called my youngest brother and told him what was going on and had him take her to a clinic in Berkeley who referred her to Alta Bates hospital. This became another issue, because now I had to go as well. He brought my mom to my job site. Mom had to use the restroom, so I told him to take her over to the elementary school's restroom because it was larger, more appropriate for adults. I got permission from the office personnel for this. What I didn't expect was for him to leave her there, now I'm getting a call from the office telling me that my mom is waiting outside the bathroom for me, sitting alone! OMG, I was so irritated.

I got mom from the office, put her in the care and drove her to the hospital. The doctors ran all kinds of test on her. I had called my niece to let her know and she called her mom to let her know. Later that evening while we were all in the waiting room, waiting for the test results, my brother thought it was a great idea to questioned the doctor about why it was taking so long and told him that he has to go home to prepare for work the next day. I'm sitting there feeling embarrassed and decided to tell him that he wasn't the only one that had to go to work the next day, but If it was so important for him to leave then he could do so and he could take my sister with him since she wasn't being helpful either. My sister got pissed off and came charging towards me like a bronco bull. I was sitting down and when I saw her coming towards me, I lifted my right leg up level with the height of the chair to prevent her from coming any closer to me.

My sister, of course lied and stated that I actually kicked her. There was a lot of loud voices in there and that brought it to the attention of the guard on duty. He was about to order us out of the hospital until I explained that there wasn't any fighting going on. My brother and sister left the hospital, but my sister decided to call her youngest daughter and tell her that same lie that I kicked her. I told her exactly what happened and that if I wanted to kick her mom, I would have stood up so I could have some power to my kick, it would not be very pro active while in a sitting position. Not to mention that my purpose there, in the hospital was to assist my ailing mother, vs fighting with her mother.

One more issue to deal with:

One day I received a call from the administrator of the building that we were living in, stating that there had been a flood in the apartment we lived in as well as the apartment below us, and the administrator also let me know that she had called Adult Protective Services, better known as APS, on me. She spoke to me in an harsh, angry tone, as if she believed that I was the reason the flood had occurred. When I asked her, "Why did she call APS, she stated in a very sharp voice, "I'll talk to you about that when you get here!" I was really blown away. This woman was very unprofessional and it made the whole process of packing up and moving a bit difficult. She told me that she wasn't going to do anything to assist us. She didn't offer another empty apartment, which I was later informed that she was supposed to do. Thank God I had the good sense to purchase renter's insurance. With this insurance, everything in mom's apartment was covered! We had people there to help me pack, and remove our things. During all the packing, I had to take my mom to various friend's homes to stay while I went back to finish packing and sleeping, in all the dampness from the flooding. I was so exhausted, sleeping very little, wondering where I was going to take my mom next, because she could only stay for a day or two at these different people's homes. The furthest place she was able to go to was in Tracy, CA, which is approximately 45 minutes to an hour away to my friend Lucy's house (who is now deceased), depending on the traffic. This was a nightmare! Once I was finally packed up, we were put in a nice Hotel in Emeryville, CA. The service there was fantastic, and we were very comfortable there. It was like a little apartment. We had a great complimentary breakfast each morning, and the staff were so accommodating, especially to my mom. I am so grateful to the staff there.

A few weeks later, I had to pack up again to move to our temporary apartment in San Leandro, CA. This was on the third floor, with a small, antiquated elevator. Although the parking space was right downstairs, the walk from the car to elevator was a long walk for mom because she couldn't walk up the stairs, we had to walk the long way around to get to the elevator, and once out of it, we had to walk back around to where we started but three floors above. Mom cried, and yelled the whole way to the front door, that she didn't want to be there. (Remember, change isn't good, especially when they don't want to do something – we didn't have this problem going to the hotel though, lol)

It took a couple of weeks at least for mom to be okay with living in the apartment. This of course was only after, Aunti and my friends who came to visit, spoke so highly of the place. I'm thinking, really mom…, it took all these other people to confirm that the apartment was cool…

Mom's condition was starting to decline while in the temporary apartment. Some of that could possibly be contributed to her feelings of isolation, being away from familiar people and not being able to walk around to her friend's apartment. I would find her not able to eat things like her vegetables, and rice without it falling onto the floor. I would literally have to either cover the floor with paper or just sweep up the spillage after she was finished eating. I had stopped giving her food that she couldn't easily pick up with her spoon (I had stopped giving her a fork). It was better for the both of us. Then there were the days that she didn't want the food that I had prepared. Sometimes, we had leftovers from food she had asked me to cook for her, but on some days, she complained to others that I had given **her some damned, old food!**

Most of her days, as I've mentioned earlier, was spent watching the television (TV). She would wake me up to turn the TV on. Every few hours during the day, I would call me to "fix" the TV because it wasn't showing her program. She didn't know that the TV had gone into sleep mode, since she had been watching the same channel most of the day. Most times, she wasn't able to change the channel, or maneuver any of the buttons. If someone called and said a certain program was on, usually my Aunti, then she would have me come and put it on that channel instead of trying to do it herself. I had already been told by her social worker not to do anything for her that she could do herself. It was just easier for her to have me to do it. This was stressful for us both.

She began losing her ability to get to the bathroom to urinate, therefore urinating all over the floor while going into the bathroom. I had to constantly disinfect the entire bathroom and surrounding areas throughout the day and night. Never, ever would I walk into the bathroom without my shoes on; there could be feces on the floor, wall, shower curtain, etc. I was so frustrated, tired, angry on one side, then I was depressed, crying daily, praying to God, asking Him why had this happen to my mom? One minute I'm so angry with her, then the next minute, I'm feeling sorry for her, knowing that this "Thing" has had a tremendous affect on her as well. I don't know, who has been affected more – her or me. I know one thing for sure, I LOVE MY MOM MORE THAN MUCH! She has been a true "Blessing" to me in more ways than I can describe. I prayed that she would have peace and joy for the rest of her days.

I got notified of my mom and I being able to move back into her apartment, I was troubled, not wanting to go back there, but I did not have a job that would take care of our living expenses, so with no other choice I had to return, dealing with another nightmare. The movers broke some of our items. I had to complete more forms, itemizing all items that were damaged. I have some issues with my own tissues, so packing/moving is an extremely difficult task for me.

Lack of Response
When Dealing with
Hospital Personnel

Soon after we moved back home, I finally had to deal with the reality that I could no longer physically, or emotionally, take care of my mom alone. I was just worn down, never able to do simple things for either of us without concern for her safety.

I decided to take my mom to a facility in San Leandro, CA around midnight, only because it was closer. Once there, I informed the intake technician that my mom was falling a lot and I *needed* her to be examined and admitted into a facility, that would be able to help her get rehabilitated. One of the nurses told me that I should go home to rest, come back in the morning since it will take a while before the doctors will know what's going on. Hours later, I received a call from a woman that identified herself as the social worker. She was asking a lot of questions, trying to find out some family history, including if I was getting any assistance from my siblings, which I told her that unfortunately, I was all alone in this situation. She then stated that my mom would be released to go home. I was shocked, angry, and confused. I told her that I had brought my mom there because I could no longer handle the needs that she had. The social worker got really irritated, raised her voice and said, "She's your mother!", as if I didn't know that. "I" was the one person who has been taking care of my mother and now I know I can't do it any longer. She said she would call me back. She never did, but she apparently spoke to one of my younger family members and she called to notify me that the hospital was calling a family meeting. I was still tired and, in my feelings, so I'm telling her, "They can't force me to have a family meeting". My niece works in the medical field, and stated, "yes they can". So, begrudgingly, I got up and went back to the hospital, where I met with other supporting family members which included my daughter. I went in to speak with the social worker who had called me earlier, and another lady, who was warm and inviting. I explained that I was told I had to come for a family meeting, and I wanted to be clear that no one in this family has been caring for my mom but myself. I also, wanted the two women to know that my siblings are going to throw daggers at me, claiming that I don't keep them informed about my mom, which is the only truth that you will hear. If they had been doing their part, then they would have been in the loop.

Well, needless to say, five minutes into the meeting, my sister started off the meeting talking about me in the third person like I was not even in the room! All due to being upset about me having Power of Attorney over my mom's medical and financial business. The funny thing is, no one was ever interested in planning to assist me with my mother, but apparently, they wanted to have authority to make decisions, wow! I just look over to the social worker, she looked at me, with the "I told you so look on my face".

My child was getting pretty upset at the things that were being said about me, which lead to some short words, like, "Don't do that" between a couple of the younger family members. I walked them out of the room and the beautiful thing about this one family member is that she apologized for coming off the wrong way, and she and my child were able to quash a situation that could have potentially blown up and ended differently, if they weren't two intelligent young ladies. I'm really proud of both of them!

Despite my feelings about the situation, the hospital released my mom to go back home. I was so depressed, because, I am now trying to figure out what to do. Fortunately, mom's social worker at an East Oakland Medical Center, called me with concerns a couple days later about mom being at the hospital. I asked her how did she know that? She said, "Because your mom is my client, I am notified whenever anything is happening with her". After telling her what happened, she stated that this hospital should have NEVER discharged my mom before finding her a rehabilitation place for her to go to. She further stated that if this ever happened again, I should notify Adult Protective Services (APS), because that's definitely classified as abuse. This was a "WOW" factor for me, because I never knew that calling them was an option for me. This made me feel a little bit more empowered.

I was quickly realizing that the day had come that I would have to make the decision to admit my mother into a facility. I had been looking around for a couple of years, so I could get her on a waiting list. Every facility that I went to, told me that she would have to be admitted from the hospital. There wasn't anything medically wrong with my mom that would constitute her being admitted – she hadn't falling, broke anything, no high blood pressure, not a thing that would constitute being hospitalized. I was so weary of being told this each time I made a phone call or drove out to the facility. I began to believe that I wouldn't ever get her the help that she and I both needed.

Approximately, one week later, I called my daughter to come and assist me in taking my mom to a hospital in Berkeley, CA. Once we arrived, two men quickly met us and asked if we needed a wheel chair and I said yes. They came back with one and sweetly helped my mom into the chair and wheeled her inside. Once I explained to the intake technician why I had brought my mom there, and as she was being seen, a really nice social worker came in and spoke to me, stating that she will definitely do everything to help me, because it is obvious that I could no longer handle the needs of my mom alone. She told me to just be patient and she would make some phone calls, that it may take a while. I must say that before I reached my daughter in the waiting room, I received a call from a woman from a Nursing Center in San Pablo, CA, stating that she had an available bed for a female! Wow, I was so happy for the both of us – mom and me!

Mom had been told about the move from some hospital personnel, before I returned to her room, and she was really upset and crying. I tried to comfort her and told her that she needed more help than I could give her and that I would be coming to see her often. We had had many discussions about her going into a facility one day, beginning when my children were very young. She actually was the one who brought up the subject, stating that if she ever needed to go into a facility, she would be okay with it, but as we all know, that always sound great until you are really faced with doing it.

She was really concerned about her friends not knowing where she was. I assured her that I would definitely let all her friends and family know where she would be.

When I texted my family to notify them that mom was now in a facility, I got some terrible responses back. I was accused of putting my mom in a less than adequate place, too far from everyone, what about her TV? you know she loves to watch TV, (this is just the next day, and again, I wasn't hearing, what can I do to help?) etc. I was told that I had to first speak with the head technician at the facility to find out what type and size TV was acceptable, then I had to order it because the store didn't stock 19-inch TV's, therefore, I had to order one online, then had to wait for it to be delivered to me. Once that happened, I had to take it to the facility and of course, there was no available parking, so I had to carry it alone from a block away up a slight incline. Even the smallest of things are heavy when you have to deal with body ailments, and have to walk a distance to the place, and then even further once you are inside the building.

I found it really interesting that everyone had an opinion about this, but wasn't involved in the journey, until they decided to "drop in." I will say that one of my male siblings did come over and get her from time to time, but I still had to do all her preparations and then wait for him to come. He's not the most time conscience person, especially if it's not a priority for him. Sometimes, she would be so angry and would have me call him to see where he was. Once my mom is dressed, she is ready to leave, even before her illness.

I was really hurt and angry, thinking, "how dare they?" I didn't put my mom there because I wanted to get rid of her, she needed to be there! The weeks following were really heartbreaking for both of us. I woke up the next morning in tears, when I looked at the chair she would always sit in, and now it's empty. I cried for hours, because I felt like my mom had just died. It was very painful, and I was questioning myself on whether I had done the right thing for her. My intelligent side knew I had done the right thing, but my heart wasn't ready to own that just yet.

I went to visit my Aunti one day to take back some things that my mom had of hers. I was feeling like she may not have wanted me to come over, which was a bit unnerving to say the least. Her eldest daughter was giving me the cold shoulder as well. This woman has been in my life, all of my life, excluding the first 4 years. We became neighbors when I was 4 years old. She taught me how to crochet, we put puzzles together, we had sewing time together, recently we made jewelry together, went fishing, etc. She doesn't have any red blood running from her veins to mines, but my love for her is no different then if it we were blood connected. I am closer to her than my real aunts only because I grew up with her, we have much history!

I spoke to a cousin that is closest in age to me about this, and what she said to me was hurtful. She stated that it was felt that I didn't do my due diligence to find a place that was worthy of my mother. I was shocked and temporarily speechless. When I could speak, I politely told her that I was hurt by that statement and that I really didn't care what anyone thought because I was the only one taking care of my mom, and I know I was doing the best that I could do under the circumstances. I also mentioned that I can't just take my mom into a facility, she has to be admitted, and in order for that to happen, I was constantly told that she had to be admitted from the hospital, and there has to be a space available for that to happen.

A few weeks later, I called a facility located in Alameda that I had tried to get my mom into before. This time, "Thank you Jesus!", I was told that they would be having some open beds in about three days! I was so happy to hear this because not only would it be closer, but it was near the water and my mom loved the water. It took maybe another couple of weeks, and I told my mom she would be moving closer to home, but she thought I meant she was going home – with me. When she got to the new place, she was pissed off again at me. I tried to explain to her that I only meant that she was moving to a better and closer place. It took some time for her to get acclimated at this place as well.

During one of our visits, she leaned over to me and said, "Sammar, I pray you will never get this "Thing" that I have." I replied, "Mom I hope not". It broke my heart. It's an internal hell that she's going through. It takes your dignity away, to have others wiping your behind, feeding you like a baby, dressing you, etc. (Although, she feeds herself – with her fingers though) I guess the good thing about this is that she has sweet, loving people that had come into her life that really cared, and actually showed it. I thank God for them and all my friends who were standing in the gap for us, especially during the hard times.

Mom loves to listen to music and sing along. So, I try to always come into the facility singing, "I always love my Mama, she's my special girl" … She hears me singing and lights up. It is so wonderful to bring happiness to others – especially to my mom.

Approximately, September 22, 2018, it was during the room checks since there's nothing going on in the activity room during that time. I decided to take mom to her room to eat the snack that I had brought to her. She loves to eat pork skins. While opening the bag, she started talking about a song, but couldn't remember the words. Finally, she started saying some words and I began to sing what I thought she was talking about, *"I know you want to leave me, but I refuse to let you go, if I have to beg, plead, for your sympathy, I don't mind cause you mean that much to me, Ain't too proud to beggggg, and you know it, please don't leave me gurllll, don't you know. Ain't too proud to pleaaaddddd, baby, babbyyyyy, please don't llleeaaavvee me gurl, don't you know….* I videoed her mouthing the words and put it on facebook, and so many people in boxed me saying how sweet this was, priceless, etc. I even had one of my friends tell me to put it on YouTube and see how many hits I would get. This was so nice and will always be a sweet memory. I don't know what made her think of this song, but it was sweet.

One of the things that I did not like is that mom couldn't walk, and she wasn't getting much therapy to get her back to walking on her own. So, her days were spent in a wheelchair, being transported from place to place during the day.

In terms of feeding herself, she wasn't able to use her utensils, so for her it was easier to use her fingers. Although she's right-handed, she had been using her left hand for eating and actually everything else. This started with the "Jerking" of her right hand, an issue that came with her dementia. So, I let her use her left so she can be in control of her eating. When I'm there, I like to feed her myself, which she really enjoyed.

On February 7, 2019, my daughter's birthday, I came to the nursing home one day to pay my mom's bill and found my sister in the lobby room with mom and a couple of other ladies. She wasn't any happier to see me than I was to see her. The night before, I had received a text from one of my cousins stating that her mom wasn't doing well. My aunt had dementia as well. I forwarded the text to a couple of people. Well, that's why my sister was there that day with mom because when she read that text, she thought the text was referring to our mother. She was so pissed off and told me that next time I should state that it's not our mother. I replied that if she had read the text, she would have realized it was about our aunt. It was obvious that she was so pissed because she came over there thinking that there was something wrong with our mother! Mind you, she hadn't been there in a long time!

I had brought mom some chicken nuggets and fries' - things I knew that she could pick up. My sister stated that she had just finished with lunch. I knew that, but I wanted to bring her something that I knew she liked, especially since she doesn't always like the food she's given there.

My sister began to ask me if mom cries when I leave. I said "No." She then stated that she had told the rehab people about her right wheel on the chair being loose and that they should replace it, but they told her they would see if they could fix it first. She then told me that I guess since you're in charge, you can handle it. Then, I had to count to ten because the next thing out of her mouth was that" If mom had exercised her arms like I told her before, she would be able to wheel herself around instead of me having to do it! I so damned angry with her, I asked the Lord to hold my tongue because I was not going to allow her to steal my peace or joy! Inside of myself, I was screaming! I wanted to slap the living shit out of her! How dare she open she mouth to once again make things about her, while mom was dealing with the loss of her abilities to function on her own!!! As calm as I could, I told her that due to her medical issues, it didn't matter if she had exercised or not, because none of that mattered any more ---**Denial!**

I was thinking as we were watching General Hospital one day, it is really interesting how the Soap Opera programs align their shows with actual things that are happening in the world. On this show, Sonny Corinthos's dad is dealing with dementia. Sonny is Port Charles's mob boss. Some of the issues he is dealing with are loud outbursts, wandering off, and what we call **Sundowners,** which means that when the sun goes down, he exhibits certain negative behaviors. He knows he is causing his son and family a lifestyle change, and stress from trying to care for him. One day he asked his therapist, at what point does your home stops being a home and becomes a prison. I found that question to be very relevant because when you're in a situation as the person with dementia, there is no place you can go without being taken like a child; then there's the caregiver who finds themselves imprisoned in a situation where the life they once knew, no longer exits.

When you are the caregiver, you are pretty much confined to the house to watch over your loved one(s). There's no partying with the friends, sleeping late, going to work, unless you can afford to bring in respite caregivers to give you a needed break. So, the person with Dementia is pissed, crying, throwing tantrums, and you as the caregiver, are feeling trapped and you are also throwing your own version of tantrums. People on the outside, can't or won't understand because they are not in your shoes walking down a road that seems endless.

Missed Event:

Today, September 19, 2018, I was totally late going to Crab Cove where my mom's facility had taken her for their annual picnic. The first thing that delayed me was that I had forgotten this was the day of the event, then once I realized this as the day for the event, some woman thought it was okay to park her car in front of the garage door that I needed to exit. I was trapped in there for at least 15 minutes before she returned, stating that she thought she had parked correctly – Really??? Then once I got to Alameda, I couldn't find the Crab Cove due to being given the wrong information, and not being given the exact address or a map of their exact location – I missed the whole event! Wow, my mom and both of her Activity Directors were a bit disappointed as well as myself. They were looking for me, and I was told later that a reminder had been left in her room!

I told him that I rarely go to her room since she is always in the Activities Room when I come. I had to speak with the administrator prior to this because I had actually made at least 4-5 attempts to find this place prior to this day's event to avoid this very thing. I had also expressed to him about how it had become a serious problem trying to connect to my mom via the phone. More times than not, when the front desk clerk answers the phone, I am being transferred to the nurses in her wing – (Gold Coast), they aren't answering, the portable phone is in use, or the batteries are dead. Mom's family on the East Coast is irritated because they are three hours ahead of us and it's difficult to get through. The administrator was very apologetic, stating that he has already gotten Comcast out to fix the phone problem but can't say exactly when the problem will be solved, but he did offer to pay for my gas, due to the inconvenience.

Once Mom was admitted and settled into the nursing center, I was then faced with getting my life back. I no longer was deemed a live in aide for mom since she was no longer living in her senior apartment. This meant that I would have to find another place to live. I hadn't been working for over a year with my substitute teaching job. Now, I am no longer getting paid from IHSS because I no longer work for mom. I am faced with not only no money but also no place to live. I was now in a different kind of hell. I spent days crying, searching for places to live, but how was I going to pay? I felt devastated, after taking care of mom alone, I am now truly alone, and with no place to go. All of our family is on the East coast. My job doesn't pay me enough to get a place to live in the High-priced Bay Area.

In the days to come, after I had been called back to substitute, I got hurt during my job assignment, and now it has created another problem. I was given a modified job assignment that would last for only three months on the job and three months off the job for a maximum of three times. When I'm taken off modified duty, I'm being paid a very minimum salary based on wages from the previous year. Well, we know that those previous years were spent mostly with my mom, and I wasn't working much at that time. I'm thinking, damn, I am still dealing with the effects of being a caregiver even after mom was admitted. Where do "I" go for assistance?

Now that mom was in a nursing facility, I had to find another place to live since Mom had been living in a low-income facility for seniors under HUD. They wouldn't allow me to continue living there although I was in the senior age bracket. While I am looking to find other housing, I received a call from my mom's nursing facility that my sister called to request a letter stating that our mom wouldn't ever be leaving that facility. The nurse wanted to know why and if she should provide her that request. I told her "absolutely not! Do not give anyone anything without my permission first. I thanked her for calling me first instead of providing my sister with that letter. My belief is that she wanted to show the letter to the housing office where mom and I was living in order to have me evicted out of the place. It was just another one of my sister's evil deeds.

Eventually, I was told that I would need to leave, since mom was no longer there. So once again, I am moving. This time I had to move in with a colleague, I will call her Chatty and paid her the $400 she requested for a room that I wasn't given a key to, had to share part of the bedroom closet and pay additional storage fees because she didn't want all my things there. I was already paying storage fees of $250+ for my things I brought back from my home in Georgia. Now I added another small storage bringing my bill to $325 per month. I have prayed, cried, then prayed again, but I still find doors closing on me. At this time, I was 62 years old and social security isn't enough, my retirement isn't enough, and now, I have a work injury and so far, I can't find a job description within my work limitations that doesn't prevent me from losing my worker's compensation case.

This chick, Chatty, apparently thought that I was there to be her companion and cook food for her, not including waiting for repair persons. Don't get it twisted, I don't mind helping, and I love cooking; I just wanted to have a place to lay my head and get "Me" together for once since I returned to the Bay Area, without thought of taking care of someone else's wants. I was truly honest with her from the beginning, telling her before I moved in that I have never lived with anyone outside of my family and was really embarrassed at having to move in with her or anyone else. I felt defeated after all my accomplishments in life, now needing to find refuge in a person's home that I didn't even know that well.

Two months later, I had told this colleague that my modified duty was ending a week prior to her coming to me stating that at the beginning of the next month, she will need to get an additional $200 from me. I can truly say that I was speechless. All I could utter out of my mouth was that I can't afford that. I was so shocked that I couldn't even look at her for at least two weeks. I called the colleague/friend, Diva #3, who had referred her to me, and she basically stated that she didn't want to be in the middle and that I should just talk to her, and she knows that she will listen. My pride had been stomped on so many times; my fear of rejection was increasing, my ability to trust people who had stated they wanted to help me was like walking on a tight rope. I didn't know who I could trust or if I should trust them.

I finally went back to Chatty's home to have this discussion with her. She assumed that I had gotten angry and should have spoken with her. Now I was thinking that she's an educated woman, she was told my situation just last week, so what was there for me to say??? I'm in her home, for reasons known to her; she knows that I was just taken off my modified duty and that meant less money that I would be receiving. The point was not that I was angry, the point was that you never once considered that I just told you that I will not be working, therefore, I will not have more money, but instead less money. So how on earth, did you fix your mouth to ask me such a thing! What I felt was "Betrayed, not believing that she really wanted to help me, but just wanting to help herself.

My Personal Thoughts

I often sit in my quiet, wondering about the why's of my journey. I wonder why I was saddled with the lonely care of my mom; why is it that my siblings felt no need to commit to the care of the woman they claimed to love. I've been told more than once by two of my siblings, that since I was living with her, I will automatically be expected to do more for mom. I have tried to understand, but I don't have any understanding of children not stepping up and actively sharing the responsibilities of their parent(s).

We were all born into this world to the same two parents, raised under the same roof, same food received, same rules to govern each of us, and the same opportunities. Being the oldest child, I was and still am expected to "keep things straight, and in line." I didn't ask for this ginormous duty, nor did I ever think that I would be the "chosen one" to fix almost all things family. Don't get this twisted; I LOVE my family, it's just that I don't always LIKE them. This world we live in is very cruel, and I just wanted for us to be more loving and flexible. Now I don't mean flexible in a way that suggests that anyone can do or say what they want to without a thought about another's feelings. I feel this incredible weight that comes with being the firstborn child. I'm expected to make everything alright for everyone. It's really exhausting because at the end of the day, who's there's to make all things good for me???

Approximately 20 years ago, while speaking to a therapist, the light bulb came on once she stated this very thing. I started tearing up because I knew then, what I hadn't realized until that conversation – I'm there for EVERYONE, but NO ONE is there for ME. Twenty years plus later, I haven't seen a real difference, until now. It actually feels worse, because our family has been challenged and is divided more so than ever before. I believe that this family division will change eventually - at least I hope so.

I'm trying to keep my sanity and still be who God wants me to be. Although I don't always understand the path, He has put me on, I try to be the best person that I can be within the confines of what I have been given. Is turning the other cheek relevant, or not? I have said, I only have two cheeks, and I've already used both, so what am I supposed to do now? It's a metaphor that I'm always trying to understand. I feel as though I'm always on this journey, trying to prove myself, or get approval from those I may think matter to me. But as I look over my life, I have come to know that the only approval I need is God's approval, but yet I feel that I fall short of that also. So, I go through life trying to do and be the best I can be, as a God-fearing human being.

Life, for me has been a bed of many changing things, specifically, since I made the decision to relocate to Georgia. I've had heartbreaking trials, I've put trust in those who claimed to love and care for me, but actually had hidden agendas which resulted in unexpected losses that I have not recovered from... We as human beings need to step aside of self and check out the bigger picture. In my world, I am always the one to put others ahead of myself. I don't do that to achieve being hailed to; I do it because someone is in need. While there are some opinions that someone may not be deserving of my assistance, I may believe in the cause.

The End of Mom's and My Journey Together

Mom had always tested Covid 19 negative when the other patients were exposed, but this last time in January 2020, when she was supposed to be quarantined, she had been exposed. She then got pneumonia two days before returning to her regular room. Yes, on her 12th quarantined day! I had already written a long letter to the Ombudsman office, because a year prior, I had made several attempts to get help from them and nothing happened. Now I was being told that a different office was handling the complaints regarding the negligence of my mom's care before Covid-19.

For a long time, no one could come inside the nursing facility anymore, making me really stressed about my mother's care. Now, I can't pop in to see what exactly is going on with her. I started noticing a decline in her attitude. She wasn't happy not being able to see me as she had become accustomed to. I couldn't see how she was, how her room looked, the type of food she was given, or the type of care givers assigned to her.

After Covid, mom had dropped from 141 pounds in December, down to 118 January 2021. I made the decision to have her go to the local general hospital. I initially met with the head doctor who I didn't like on sight due to his lack of compassion or bedside manner. He didn't act like a doctor who was concerned for a dementia woman that had contracted this horrible virus through no means of her own. She was at the mercy of people, who were put in charge of keeping her safe and they failed. The head doctor basically told me this: you have two paths to go – either you give her a feeding tube or put her in hospice! I felt like slapping him. How dare he be so uncaring when he took an oath to do no harm! I really had nothing more to say to him at that point other than, I want to see my mother. He took me to her room and stayed there for the few minutes he said I was allowed to be there, which he said was fifteen (15) minutes. I wasn't in the room but maybe half of that time. The only good thing that came out of that meeting was the fact that the doctor witnessed my mother drinking from a straw for me and speaking to me, answering me saying, "yes baby", and telling me she loved me. I said, "Did you see that, did you hear that?" He said no he hadn't until I came there.

It took many conversations with different hospital personnel including the Palliative Care unit before I was able to get the permission to visit my mom in the hospital. I was told that I could only visit for an hour or so, but I was there the next day for five hours! We both had a great time, laughing and singing. One of the nurses came in to see who was singing. We were so loud, but the nurse was loving it and said it was nice to see mom in good spirits.

After countless conversations with back-and-forth thoughts of whether I was going through with having a feeding tube put into my mother's stomach, on the 13th hour, the doctor call me the night before the scheduled operation, stating that it had been decided that there would be no surgery for my mother. Initially, I was very angry to hear this, at the same time, I was actually relieved. I say this because I never really wanted surgery for her. I was only considering this option due to the fact that she was not eating enough to sustain her life, and I wanted her to live.

Once it was decided that the surgery was off, I had to now make another decision – was I going to put her in hospice? I knew that this didn't mean she was being given X amount of time to live, but instead, it would give her more care and it would give me more eyes watching over her once she was taken back to her nursing facility. My decision to have her put into hospice care was the best thing that I could have done for mom at that time. This afforded me and everyone else who loved her to finally be "*allowed*" to come into the nursing home and visit with her, even though other patients weren't allowed visitors. It's funny how being close to death will change all previous medical do's and don'ts 's or can and can't rules. This of course allowed my family members and her close friend and co-worker, the opportunity to see her one more time.

The youngest of my family members who hadn't seen mom for a long time, was simply devastated. He couldn't believe his eyes. I knew and said long before that this would be the case. He didn't want to deal with the process and now this process was dealing with him. The same goes for the 1st born brother. The only difference was that he had been in and out of the prison system so he couldn't come to visit, although, I had written him countless times trying to educate him on the disposition of our mother. He was always unnerved when he actually saw her. Not believing that this thing called "Dementia" was slowly killing his mother. He instead preferred to believe that the workers at the nursing home was "Doing something" to his mother.

The other brother could only sit crying quietly. He really doesn't know how to deal with things like this. I don't say this to excuse him not coming to see her more often, but it just sad to me that no one can stand up, and take some responsibility but me. My sister would come rarely as well, and when she did, she had complaints that she shared with me a year and a month prior to mom's passing. These complaints weren't as much about our mother, as it was about her, and how she couldn't handle doing things like pushing mom's wheelchair into the lobby (when she could have asked someone there for assistance), or asked me, "Does mom cry when you leave? These were some of the things she mentioned the last time I saw her. I remember that I was so angry at her for once again, making all things about her!

I'm so grateful that all of mom's children, grandchildren and great grandson was given the opportunity to visit her right before she passed. I of course felt bad because she didn't get to see my granddaughters, one of which was the youngest and mom had only seen her on a video and pictures. I know we all have to leave this earth one day. It's never known when, because our Lord and Savior is the only one to make that decision, but Covid-19 is the reason for us losing our dear sweetly beloved mother sooner, before dementia could take her away. For me, this lost is GREAT! I know the rest of my siblings are dealing with their lost in a much different way than me.

I will cherish all the fun and crazy memories that I couldn't possibly put in one book at this time, but *Erlene* is surely missed and for me there is a gaping hole in my heart, and I don't know just yet, how I will be able to fill it – maybe never…

I am now trying to pick up the pieces of my life and it isn't easy. I have multiple body pains from a life of working with the special needs' population, adults as well as small children and ending with my mom. I truly feel as though I'm in a place of uncertainty, I'm now dealing with all things Medicare and trying to find a new a path of employment, knowing that at my age, although I'm educated, this education can and has been a negative when applying for jobs. It has been so long since I've had to apply for a job, and nothing is done the way that I once knew! Doing everything virtually is a huge hindrance. How are employers supposed to notice me out of the thousands applying on the web? But everything I try to do is affected by my health and needing to first be retrained. Damn, I'm already 65, how much time will pass before I can get reacclimated! Now add all my ailments from worker's compensation…Nothing is really going right for me to be a self-reliant woman that I once was. Was this supposed to happen this way? I find myself wondering Why, what if…

On **Friday, February 26, 2021**, at 5:15a, the Lord gave Mom her wings as some would say. As soon as the phone ranged, the name of her nursing home showed up. I knew the news would not be favorable. I had tossed and turned all night long in my bed at the hotel in Fresno, California. I had driven down there the day before to support one of my friends at the memorial for her nephew. I was so hurt at hearing this but was also very angry at the attitudes of personnel who was urging me to get her removed from their facility within a four-hour period. I felt threatened, because the social worker literally told me that if I didn't get her body removed in the 4-hour window post death, it would be done for me at my expense! Mind you, I am in another city, and it is before business hours. Social services are supposed to be there to **"Support"** not to", **"Threaten** which is how I felt. My mom died alone and I can only believe that she went peacefully in her sleep.

This has actually been the hardest book I've ever written. It has been three years in the making and I still find myself wondering if I have covered all the important aspects of my journey. It seems that I may have to possibly do a part two, in order to enlighten and share more about the aftermath of this journey, because some people seem to believe that once your love one passes over, this is the end, but that is not true. This is actually the beginning of the rebuilding process for the caregiver...But, before I do that, I now work at a nursing facility and I'm now seeing things from the back end. I am not happy at all the things that I have witnessed, but at the same time I feel for both sides of this coin. What I don't understand, is how working all your life, giving yourself to a job for most of us and ending up needing someone else to care for you and fighting for the right to live your last days with self-respect. Medicare is a beast, not knowing how to matriculate within their system is mind blowing to the best of us. No one should have to struggle for medical care, but that is a true issue in this America. How to change it is the question. The United States residents are more concerned about animals that they are about people of any age. I just wish that we, the people, would put our fight for the elderly who becomes fragile in many ways; some who have no family to care for them, and some have relatives that refuses to care. I pray that this mindset changes, and we all choose to do the right thing for the people who once sacrificed everything for us.

True Reflections

Sitting here reflecting on conversations I have been having much too frequently of late. Having conversations with family, friends, church family, even random people along the way. It seems there's a number of us who are dealing with a loved one who is experiencing symptoms associated with Dementia/Alzheimer's, either directly or indirectly. During my conversations with various people in and out of the medical arena that every 66 seconds that someone develops Dementia, this life draining disease. Not good! How did it get to this alarming rate?

Do doctors really know the difference or are they just speculating? Why does it take so long to receive a diagnosis for it? If the patient is showing signs and, has a family health history of the disease, why must it get to the extreme stages before a diagnosis is given?

There are medications available so we're told, however, they may be unreliable. In fact, they may even turn out to be harmful; so, we're told. Wow!

So, what do you say when your loved one asks, "What's wrong with me, I can't remember anything?"

Hmmm, remember what Dad had, and Aunt so and so, or your sibling?

One of my aunts always stated, I been kno'd that she or he had that STUFF (That's the way she speaks). Well, it might be the same thing, but I can tell you that you will get to the point where you can't remember how to get to the bathroom, and once you get there, you're not quite sure what to do.

How do we tell them there are things they absolutely have to get in order very soon, if we can't really tell them why because, we may be just speculating? They're confused and we're confused as well.

How do we ease their fears and calm them about their anxieties regarding memory loss, delusions, helplessness, and sleeplessness? What do we say, what do we do? Each one, teach one I guess; as we've been doing through our conversations.

Loved ones who become caregivers WANT to know, NEED to know, and DESERVE to have more information going forward with this dreaded disease. We must prepare our loved ones as well as ourselves, and in order to do that, WE must be better informed.

Other People's Account of Their Experiences with Their Family Member's Journey...

What are some issues that were experienced in my loved ones with Dementia, (earlier signs)?

- *Short-term memory problems (misplacing everyday items often)*
- *Losing directions previously known*
- *Misplacing clothing or jewelry and accusing others of removing it*
- *Forgetting and/or misdialing phone numbers constantly*
- *Experiencing delusions and/or hallucinations*
- *Sleeplessness*
- *Loss of appetite or excessive eating*
- *Losing touch with reality, (thinking TV personalities are speaking specifically to them*
- *Aggressiveness*
- *A tendency of combativeness*
- *DC of Oakland*

◊ *The doctors would not listen when family expressed major concerns about Mrs. Cecile exhibiting certain symptoms. The doctor said she was okay based on her word. As a result of her behavior, her husband moved out and she had unfounded distrust in her daughter and granddaughter. This left Mrs. Cecile alone in her home and not taking prescribed meds, thereby leading to further strokes, blindness etc. This was also a safety issue for her. She was admitted to one facility, and she called police on them, and they released her. Adult Services was called into the home and other interventions – all to no avail.*

PR, Oakland, CA

◊   *I would say it's hard because you never get a break from it.
And that's probably why I like to leave home a lot. It's like one
day I went from loving to come home from school to hating it,
because I no longer have a choice or say so on how I live my life.
I personally limit myself from everything to keep everybody else
happy. Such as, not doing any after-school activities because I
need to be home in time, so my mom doesn't have to deal with
both me and my grandmother. Which puts me in a place where
I have to also handle all my teenage emotions on my own and
having no one to run to and being afraid that one day you
won't be able to handle it all and might burst and you can't even
explain that because you don't want to be a burden. I no longer
feel like my mom's baby girl or my mom's first priority. Now I
feel as if there's no time for me so I shouldn't even bother to ask
or say anything. And there's really no point in saying how much
I hate it here because nothing will change which adds onto the
hill of emotions built up waiting on the day to burst.*

T.R. – Oakland Youth

◊   *One sunny morning while shopping for fresh veggies for mom,
I was told that one of the ladies in the room was trying to get
my attention. I didn't know the lady, but she definitely had
something to say to me. She began by saying that she wanted to
tell me that she watches me as I walk to the car and back with
my mom and that she appreciates how I don't hold her hand, but
let her walk alone, staying near her in case she needs any help.
She went on to say that she doesn't know why she's crying, but*

it's wonderful to see someone doing for their parent what she witnesses me doing because that's a rare thing in their building. This lady doesn't know to this day how much joy she gave me that day. It's funny how you think that no one notices the little things you do, and this happens. I always say that we NEVER know who's watching. I will always appreciate and cherish her words forever!

Divajek – Oakland

It is now December 26, 2021. It has been ten (10) months since my sweet mom has transitioned form this place. I am still not understanding it all. A year ago, mom tested positive for Covid-19, she was transferred into yet another wing of the nursing home to ISOLATED again! We all know that isolation is not a good thing for anyone, especially people with dementia. I have so many issues with this. 1. She contracted this horrible illness from someone who worked in that facility – she wasn't going out for any reason, not to a doctor's appointment – nothing! After everything this lady had gone through – now this! I can't blame her passing on dementia at this point because until she got Covid-19 she was doing okay. But having this on top of dementia further escalated her inability to swallow, her non desire for food – the inability to thrive is what the medical profession would say, which we know was coming at some point, but Covid-19???Where in the Hell did this come from???…

I would like to leave you, my readers with some golden nuggets-

It's important to know that it's really okay to feel disappointed about the way life has turned out for you; don't beat yourself down for feeling this way. Some examples: Why can't I utilize the degrees that I have studied and worked so hard for...Why shouldn't I feel bad when the roof over my head doesn't belong to me? These things make me "feel less than". Why am I the only person giving up their time and energy to help their loved one?

* Your childhood, be it good or bad, will affect you for the rest of your life, but for every bad thing that happens, something good will always come from it.

* It's okay to own your feelings, and others should allow you to do so without giving you their so-called opinion. At the end of the day, The Bumpy Roads Can Be Smoothed and You Can ALWAYS Change Your Lane – Nothing stays the same forever... Amen!

REFERENCES

*Info gotten from ActiveBeat, written by Anna June 10, 2013

(P. Ford-Martin 2020)- reviewed medically by Jennifer Casarella, MD 2020

Online References

https://www.dementia.org/dementia-pugilistica

www.ingramcontent.com/pod-product-compliance
Lightning Source LLC
Chambersburg PA
CBHW021509210526
45463CB00002B/958